First Aid in Neurology: Emergency Response and Care

First Aid in Neurology: Emergency Response and Care

Dr. Khushboo Gupta
Assistant Professor
Trilok Singh TT College
Lakshmangarh, Sikar
Rajasthan, India

HEMAKSHEE PUBLICATION

First Aid in Neurology: Emergency Response and Care

Edition: 2026
ISBN (paperback): 978-93-48873-49-1

Published by Hemakshee Publication

HEMAKSHEE PUBLICATION

Sikar, Rajasthan, India

Email: support@hemaksheepublication.com

Website: www.hemaksheepublication.com

Contents

Part III: First Aid Techniques and Tools

Part IV: Special Situations and Preventive Measures

Preface

Neurological conditions are no longer confined to hospital settings—they emerge suddenly, at home, on the road, or in schools. Despite this, public knowledge about managing such emergencies remains limited. As a healthcare educator, I've witnessed many lives affected not just by the illness itself—but by the delay in recognizing it.

This book is born out of a deep need for community-level neurological awareness. It simplifies science without losing accuracy. The structure is deliberately action-focused—with flowcharts, tables, checklists, and emergency guides. Whether you're a caregiver for someone with epilepsy, a teacher seeing a child faint, or a good Samaritan witnessing a roadside injury—this guide is for you.

Let this book be a bridge between fear and confidence, panic and purpose.

— Dr. Khushboo Gupta

Biography

(Dr. Khushboo Gupta)

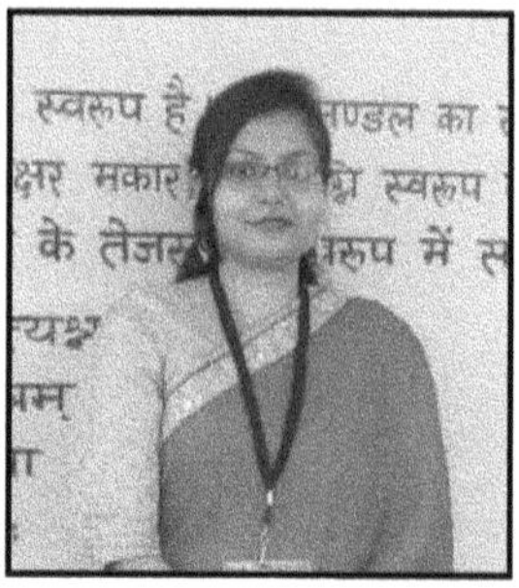

Dr. Khushboo Gupta is a PhD Home Science (Food Science and Nutrition) from Banasthali Vidyapith, Newai, India. She has been teaching subject including food chemistry, food analysis, therapeutic nutrition, human nutrition, human physiology and community nutrition, etc. Presently she is working as Assistant Professor in Trilok Singh TT College, Laxmangarh, Sikar, Rajasthan.

She is MSc Gold medalist and had **cleared UGC-NET and RPSC-SET examination.** Dr Gupta holds Advance Diploma in French Language from Banasthali Vidyapith; Diploma in Naturopathy and Yoga (NDDY) from Gandhi Smarak Prakritik Chikitsa Samiti (Regd.), New Delhi; Certificate in Homeopathic Medicinal System conducted by Vardhman Mahaveer Open University, Kota and Certificate in Statistical Techniques and Applications. She has featured in several programs of All India Radio and Radio Banasthali (FM 90.4).

Dr. Khushboo is actively involved in community activities especially those concerned with self-employment, health and wellness, optimum nutrition and how to improve quality of life of a person and family. She is the keynote speaker and founder of her YouTube channel "Khushboo

Health Care" through which she provides education related to optimum health, wellness and nutrition to masses. Dr. Gupta has published about more than 30 research papers in reputed national and international journals; 22 book chapters in different edited books, several news paper and magazine articles related to health, nutrition and new food product formulation. She authored three books related to elderly nutrition and financial management; edited **twenty eight** books related to community science, food science and nutrition, health and wellness, issues with girls, health for all, sustainable development, food safety and security, breastfeeding, skill inculcation, Inflammatory bowel disease, millets and celiac disease for upliftment of the individuals of the society. She presented her research work in more than 26 national and international conferences. Her research is primarily in the area of food processing entrepreneurial skill Inculcation and geriatric nutrition. **The patent office, Government of India has granted a patent to Dr. Khushboo for her research on food formulation using RSM.** Dr. Gupta has successfully completed more than 30 courses on various diverse topics organized by SWAYAM, UNICEF, WHO and Cornell University.

In past she had worked as Assistant Professor (Food and Nutrition) in Modi University, Laxmangarh, Sikar; worked as Master Trainer in Agriculture University, Kota. During her PhD she had worked as UGC- SRF in Banasthali Vidyapith, Newai. One feather in her cap is that she had worked as regular trainee dietitian in dietetics department of Post Graduate Institute of Medical Education and Research (PGIMER), Chandigarh and got her short-term attachment certificate. She won many awards in different seminars and conferences for her contribution in scientific world. Apart from them, she is rewarded with **Teacher Honour award** by

Lions Club Kota South (September, 2017); '**Award of Honour**' given by All Rajasthan Qualified Homoeopathic Doctors Association in Homoeopathic Scientific Seminar, 2017, **Excellence Academician Award** given by Akhil Bhartiya Agrawal Mahasabha (Reg), Kota Branch (2023) and **Shakti Vandan Award** given by S.R.S.T. College of Education Ova Jahanabad, Bihar in association with Kalindi Prakashan, Ajamgarh, UP (2024).

She is the life member of many reputed institutes i.e. Nutrition Society of India, Indian Dietetic Association, The Indian Science Congress Association and Institute of Scholars and giving her services for upliftment of community.

Chapter 1
Introduction to Neurological First Aid

The Urgency of Neurological Emergencies

Neurological emergencies are among the most frightening and time-sensitive medical situations. Unlike external wounds or fractures, injuries to the brain, spinal cord, or nervous system often have no visible signs—but they can cause sudden unconsciousness, seizures, paralysis, and even death within minutes. These emergencies demand rapid recognition and an immediate, informed response.

Neurological conditions such as **stroke**, **seizures**, **head trauma**, or **spinal cord injury** require **"golden hour" intervention**. The faster the response, the higher the chances of survival and recovery without permanent disability. This highlights the importance of **first aid knowledge specific to neurology**—a domain often overlooked in conventional first aid training.

Why Neurological First Aid is Different

Most people are trained in general first aid—like treating wounds, choking, or heart attacks—but few are equipped to deal with the complexities of neurological events. Here's how neurological first aid differs:

- **Symptoms are subtle or invisible:** A stroke may look like simple confusion or facial asymmetry; a brain injury might present as mild dizziness initially.

- **Time is critical but deceptive:** In neurological cases, even if symptoms seem mild, irreversible damage may already be happening.
- **The margin of error is small:** Inappropriate handling (such as moving a spinal injury patient) can worsen the outcome dramatically.

Goals of Neurological First Aid

1. **Rapid Identification** of warning signs like slurred speech, loss of balance, or seizures.
2. **Prevention of Further Harm** by avoiding unnecessary movements and providing basic support.
3. **Timely Activation of Emergency Services** and proper reporting of symptoms.
4. **Supportive Care** until professional medical help arrives, including protection from aspiration during seizures, or maintaining airway in unconscious patients.

Who Should Read This Book?

This book is intended for:

- **General Public**: Parents, teachers, caregivers, and community workers
- **Medical and Paramedical Students**: Looking for a focused approach on neurological first response

- **Rural Healthcare Volunteers**: Where quick transport to hospitals may be difficult
- **School and College Staff**: Often the first responders to student fainting or seizures
- **Anyone with Family History of Stroke, Epilepsy, or Brain Injury**

Common Myths and Facts

Myth	Fact
Wait for seizures to stop before calling help	Seizures lasting more than 5 minutes are life-threatening. Act fast.
Stroke only affects the elderly	It can affect young people too. Even children.
Giving water to a fainting person helps	Can cause choking. Wait until they are fully conscious.
A head injury is fine if there's no bleeding	Internal brain injury may still occur. Observation is critical.

Chapter 2

Basic Neuroanatomy and Brain Function

Understanding the basic structure and function of the nervous system allows one to grasp the seriousness of neurological emergencies and why certain symptoms must not be ignored.

The Human Nervous System

The nervous system is the body's control center, made up of:

1. **Central Nervous System (CNS)**: Includes the brain and spinal cord.
2. **Peripheral Nervous System (PNS)**: Comprises all the nerves outside the CNS.

The nervous system controls everything—from thinking, movement, and sensation, to breathing, heart rate, and digestion.

Parts of the Brain and Their Functions

1. **Cerebrum**:
   - Largest part of the brain.
   - Divided into left and right hemispheres.
   - Controls voluntary movements, speech, vision, reasoning, memory, and emotions.

2. **Cerebellum:**
    - Located under the cerebrum.
    - Responsible for coordination, balance, and posture.
3. **Brainstem:**
    - Connects the brain to the spinal cord.
    - Controls vital functions such as heartbeat, breathing, and consciousness.
    - Damage here can be fatal.
4. **Spinal Cord:**
    - Runs from the brainstem to the lower back.
    - Transmits nerve signals between the brain and body.
    - Injury can lead to paralysis depending on the level of damage.

How Damage to These Areas Affects the Body

Area Affected	Likely Impact
Left Cerebrum	Speech loss, right-side weakness
Right Cerebrum	Visual-spatial problems, left-side weakness
Cerebellum	Poor balance, tremors
Brainstem	Irregular breathing, heart rate,

	loss of consciousness
Spinal Cord (Neck)	Quadriplegia (paralysis of all four limbs)
Spinal Cord (Lower Back)	Paraplegia (paralysis of legs only)

Chapter 3
Neurological Assessment in Emergencies

When a person shows sudden neurological symptoms, a structured assessment can help identify the severity and cause. These tools are used by both professionals and trained first responders to make immediate decisions.

1. FAST Assessment for Stroke

This is a globally accepted and simple technique to identify strokes:

- **F – Face Drooping**: Ask the person to smile. Is one side of the face drooping?
- **A – Arm Weakness**: Ask them to raise both arms. Does one arm drift downward?
- **S – Speech Difficulty**: Is their speech slurred, or are they unable to speak?
- **T – Time to Call Emergency Services**: If you see even one of these signs, act fast.

2. Glasgow Coma Scale (GCS)

Used to assess the level of consciousness in an injured or unconscious person:

Response Type	Score Range
Eye Opening	4 (Spontaneous) to 1 (None)
Verbal Response	5 (Oriented) to 1 (None)
Motor Response	6 (Obeys Commands) to 1 (None)

Interpretation:

- 13–15 = Mild brain injury
- 9–12 = Moderate injury
- ≤8 = Severe injury (needs urgent care)

3. Pupillary Reflex Check

Shine a small light into each eye:

- **Normal**: Pupil constricts quickly to light.
- **Abnormal**: One or both pupils remain dilated, sluggish, or unequal—suggesting possible brain pressure or injury.

4. Posturing in Unconscious Patients

Unusual posturing indicates severe brain injury:

- **Decorticate Posturing**: Arms flexed, legs extended → damage to cerebral cortex.
- **Decerebrate Posturing**: Arms and legs extended and rigid → brainstem damage. Both require emergency medical attention.

5. Observing Vital Signs

Vital signs may also hint at brain involvement:

- **Slow heart rate + High blood pressure**: May suggest increased intracranial pressure.
- **Abnormal breathing patterns**: Possible brainstem dysfunction.
- **Sudden rise or fall in temperature**: Could indicate infection or hypothalamic involvement.

When to Seek Emergency Care Immediately

- Sudden confusion, loss of vision, or slurred speech
- A seizure lasting more than 5 minutes
- Sudden severe headache with vomiting
- Head or spine injury after a fall or accident
- Unconsciousness or unresponsiveness

Summary of Part I: Key Concepts to Remember

Topic	Takeaway
Neurological emergencies	Require immediate, informed action
Brain functions	Knowing which part of the brain does what helps predict danger
FAST & GCS	Easy-to-use tools for recognizing strokes or injuries
Pupils & Posturing	Critical signs of brain function or deterioration
Don't wait	Time is brain—call emergency services fast

Chapter 4
Stroke

Understanding Stroke

A stroke occurs when blood flow to a part of the brain is interrupted or reduced, preventing brain tissue from getting oxygen and nutrients. Brain cells begin to die within minutes.

Types of Stroke

1. **Ischemic Stroke** (87% of all strokes)
    - Caused by a blockage (blood clot or plaque) in an artery.
2. **Hemorrhagic Stroke**
    - Caused by bleeding in or around the brain due to ruptured blood vessels.
3. **Transient Ischemic Attack (TIA)**
    - Also called a "mini-stroke." Symptoms last for a few minutes to hours and resolve, but it is a warning sign for future stroke.

Warning Signs – Use the FAST Rule

- **F – Face Drooping:** Ask the person to smile.
- **A – Arm Weakness:** Ask them to raise both arms.

- **S – Speech Difficulty**: Is their speech slurred or strange?
- **T – Time to Call Emergency Help**.

First Aid for Stroke

- Stay calm and **call emergency services immediately**.
- **Lay the person on their side** with head slightly elevated.
- **Do not give anything by mouth**, including food or drink.
- **Note the time** when symptoms began—this helps doctors decide on clot-busting treatment.
- **Keep the person warm and comfortable.**
- Monitor breathing and pulse.

Chapter 5
Seizures and Epilepsy

Understanding Seizures

Seizures occur when there is sudden, abnormal electrical activity in the brain. Causes may include epilepsy, head injury, infection, high fever (especially in children), or drug overdose.

Types of Seizures

- **Generalized tonic-clonic (grand mal)**: Full-body convulsions, loss of consciousness.
- **Absence (petit mal)**: Brief lapses in awareness.
- **Focal (partial)**: Starts in one part of the brain, may or may not affect consciousness.
- **Febrile seizures**: Common in young children during fever spikes.

First Aid During a Seizure

- **Do not panic.** Stay with the person.
- **Protect from injury:** Clear the area, cushion their head.
- **Do not hold them down or put anything in their mouth.**
- **Turn them on their side** to prevent choking on saliva or vomit.

- **Time the seizure.** If it lasts more than **5 minutes**, call emergency services.
- After the seizure, reassure the person as they regain awareness (postictal phase).

Chapter 6
Traumatic Brain Injury (TBI)

Causes

- Road traffic accidents
- Falls (especially in elderly and children)
- Sports injuries
- Physical assault

Symptoms

- Confusion or loss of consciousness
- Vomiting, headache, dizziness
- Bleeding from nose/ears
- Unequal pupils
- Seizures
- Memory loss

First Aid for Head Injury

- **Call emergency services** for any head injury with altered consciousness.
- If bleeding, apply gentle pressure with a clean cloth.
- **Do not move the person** if a spinal injury is suspected.

- **Check for breathing and pulse.** Begin CPR if necessary.
- **Do not give fluids or medications.**
- Keep them still and comfortable. Monitor for changes in consciousness.

Chapter 7
Spinal Cord Injury

Common Causes

- Car/motorcycle accidents
- Falls from height
- Diving in shallow water
- Violence or trauma

Symptoms

- Weakness or paralysis in limbs
- Loss of bladder/bowel control
- Numbness or tingling
- Severe back or neck pain
- Difficulty breathing (if upper spine is involved)

First Aid for Suspected Spinal Injury

- **Do not move the person unless absolutely necessary.**
- **Call emergency services immediately.**
- Support the **head and neck** in the position you find them.
- If CPR is needed, do it **without tilting the head back.**

- Use a **rolled towel or clothing** to keep the neck stable until help arrives.

Chapter 8
Meningitis and Encephalitis

Meningitis is inflammation of the protective membranes of the brain and spinal cord.

Encephalitis is inflammation of the brain tissue itself.

Causes

- Viral or bacterial infections
- Fungal infections (rare)
- Autoimmune conditions

Symptoms

- High fever
- Severe headache
- Stiff neck
- Vomiting
- Seizures
- Sensitivity to light
- Altered consciousness

First Aid Measures

- **Seek immediate medical attention.**
- Keep the person calm and monitor for seizures.

- If unconscious, turn to one side to prevent aspiration.
- **Do not delay.** Early treatment is essential, especially in bacterial meningitis.

Chapter 9
Migraine and Severe Headache Disorders

Migraine

- Throbbing pain usually on one side of the head
- Nausea, vomiting
- Sensitivity to light or sound
- Visual aura (in some people)

Danger Signs in Headache (Red Flags)

- Sudden, intense headache ("thunderclap headache")
- Headache with fever, stiff neck, or confusion
- Headache after a head injury
- Headache that wakes you from sleep
- Headache with weakness or seizures

First Aid for Migraine

- Help the person lie in a **quiet, dark room**.
- Apply a **cold pack** to the forehead.
- Encourage **hydration**, unless they're vomiting.
- Avoid strong smells or noise.
- **Monitor** for worsening symptoms.

If any red flags are present, **seek emergency medical care.**

Chapter 10

Fainting (Syncope) and Collapse

Causes

- Sudden drop in blood pressure
- Dehydration
- Standing up too fast
- Emotional shock
- Heart or neurological conditions

Symptoms Before Fainting

- Dizziness
- Blurred vision
- Weakness
- Nausea
- Ringing in ears

First Aid for Fainting

- **Lay the person flat on their back.**
- **Elevate the legs** to improve blood flow to the brain.
- Loosen tight clothing.
- **Do not give water** until fully conscious.

- If they don't regain consciousness in 1 minute, **call emergency services**.
- Observe for seizures, irregular breathing, or signs of stroke.

Chapter 11

Neurological Emergencies in Children

Common Neurological Emergencies in Children

- **Febrile seizures**: Seizures due to high fever, common between 6 months and 5 years.
- **Head injuries** from falls and accidents
- **Hydrocephalus complications**
- **Infections** like meningitis
- **Congenital conditions** like epilepsy

First Aid for Febrile Seizures

- **Stay calm.**
- **Place child on side** to avoid choking.
- **Remove tight clothing.**
- **Do not put anything in the mouth.**
- After seizure ends, sponge body with **lukewarm water** (not cold) to lower fever.
- **Seek pediatric care immediately**—especially if seizure lasts >5 minutes.

Key Takeaways from Part II

Emergency	Critical Action
Stroke	Use FAST, call emergency help fast
Seizure	Don't restrain, protect from injury, turn sideways
Head Injury	Keep still, monitor for vomiting, unequal pupils
Spinal Injury	Do not move, stabilize head and neck
Meningitis	Recognize fever + stiff neck + confusion
Migraine	Cold compress, dark room, avoid red flag symptoms
Fainting	Lay flat, elevate legs, observe for breathing
Febrile Seizures	Cool the child, turn on side, seek urgent care

Chapter 12

Basic Life Support (BLS) and CPR in Neurological Cases

Why BLS Matters in Neurological Emergencies

Basic Life Support (BLS) is a life-saving technique for managing victims of cardiac arrest, respiratory failure, or unconsciousness. In neurological cases, especially **stroke, seizures**, or **traumatic brain injury**, BLS plays a critical role in preventing **secondary brain damage** due to lack of oxygen.

Steps of BLS (As per American Heart Association guidelines)

A. Assess the Situation

- Ensure safety of the scene.
- Tap and shout: "Are you okay?"
- Check for **responsiveness, breathing**, and **pulse**.

B. Call for Help

- If unresponsive, **call emergency services immediately.**
- Ask someone to bring an **AED** (Automated External Defibrillator) if available.

C. Start Chest Compressions (If No Pulse)

- Place hands in the center of the chest.

- Compress **at least 2 inches deep** at a rate of **100–120 compressions per minute.**
- Allow full chest recoil between compressions.

D. Rescue Breaths

- Give 2 breaths after every 30 compressions.
- Use a barrier device if available.
- Continue until medical help arrives.

Special Notes for Neurological Cases

- In **stroke**: Maintain airway, place patient in recovery position if breathing but unconscious.
- In **seizures**: Wait till seizure ends unless the person stops breathing.
- In **head injuries**: Be cautious with neck movement; protect cervical spine during CPR.

Chapter 13

Emergency Medications and Neurological First Aid Kits

Common Emergency Medications (As Advised by Doctors Only)

Drug	Used For	Form
Midazolam/ Diazepam	Seizure control	Nasal spray, rectal gel, IV
Aspirin (300 mg)	Suspected ischemic stroke (if advised)	Tablet
Paracetamol	Fever management in children (febrile seizures)	Syrup, tablet
Mannitol (IV)	Brain swelling (hospital setting)	IV
Antiemetics	Vomiting post head injury	Tablet, injection

Note: Never administer medicines without prescription. These are handled by medical professionals.

What to Include in a Neurological First Aid Kit

- **Gloves and masks** (disposable)
- **Emergency contact card**
- **Cold packs** (for migraine or fever)
- **Flashlight** (to check pupils)
- **CPR face shield**
- **Timer or stopwatch** (to time seizures)
- **Clean cloths** or towel (for bleeding or support)
- **Notebook and pen** (for recording symptoms, times)
- **Antiseptic wipes**
- **Digital thermometer**
- **Basic pain relief medications** (if advised)

Chapter 14

Safe Transportation of Neurological Patients

Transporting a patient incorrectly can worsen spinal injuries or brain trauma. Here are steps to ensure safety.

General Transport Guidelines

- Never move a patient with **suspected spine injury** unless absolutely necessary.
- Use a **flat, firm board** or **stretcher**.
- If head injury is suspected, **immobilize the neck and head** using rolled cloth or foam.

During Transportation

- Keep the patient **lying flat** unless vomiting or unconscious—then place in **recovery position.**
- Monitor **breathing and consciousness** regularly.
- Keep the environment **calm and quiet**, especially in seizure-prone patients.
- Do not allow the patient to **walk unaided**, even if they insist.

Chapter 15
Communication During Neurological Emergencies

Why Communication Matters

In neurological emergencies, time is critical. Proper communication with emergency responders can **save time, reduce delays**, and improve care quality.

What to Report to Emergency Services

- When symptoms started (very important for stroke)
- Type and duration of seizure (if applicable)
- Any falls, injuries, or trauma
- Medications the person is on
- Known medical history (epilepsy, stroke, diabetes)
- Current consciousness level and breathing status

Effective Communication Tips

- Stay calm and speak clearly.
- Use **short, factual statements:** "The person fell. Unconscious. Seizure lasted 3 minutes. Breathing now. Not responding fully."
- If calling from a rural area, give clear **landmarks and address.**

- If trained, use **neurological terms** (e.g., decerebrate posturing, GCS score, unequal pupils).

Communicating with Family or Bystanders

- Provide **reassurance**.
- Assign roles (e.g., call ambulance, clear space, bring ID).
- If the patient is awake but confused, **do not overload with questions**.

Key Takeaways from Part III

Skill	Summary
BLS & CPR	Preserve oxygen to the brain; use carefully in neuro cases
Neuro First Aid Kit	Include basic protective, monitoring, and supportive tools
Emergency Medications	Use only under medical advice; key for seizure/stroke management
Patient Transport	Keep spine stable, avoid unnecessary movement
Communication	Report clearly to help EMS plan ahead

Chapter 16

First Aid in Rural or Resource-Limited Settings

The Challenge of Limited Resources

In rural or remote areas, access to advanced neurological care, trained professionals, or even emergency services may be delayed or unavailable. This makes **basic first aid knowledge and improvisation skills critical.**

Key Strategies for Rural Settings

□ **Use What You Have Wisely**

- **Pillows, folded clothes, or sacks** can serve as neck or head support.
- Use a **wooden plank, door, or cot** as a makeshift stretcher for spine-injured patients.
- A **mobile phone flashlight** can substitute for a pupil-check torch.

□ **Stay Calm and Follow Basics**

- Airway, Breathing, Circulation (ABC) checks come first.
- Do **not attempt to feed or medicate** unless advised.
- Avoid overcrowding around the patient.

□ **Transport Protocols**

- If transport is needed:
    - Keep the **neck and spine immobilized.**
    - Assign **one person to observe breathing/consciousness** during travel.
    - Prefer **ambulances** where available; if not, use a **flat vehicle** with padding.

Empowering Rural Communities

- **Train local volunteers** in neurological first aid.
- **Distribute posters** showing stroke and seizure signs in local languages.
- Conduct **village health camps** with practical demonstrations.

Chapter 17

Neurological First Aid During Disasters and Mass Casualties

Disasters like earthquakes, floods, building collapses, or road pile-ups can result in mass trauma, including head and spinal injuries.

Triage in Neurological Emergencies

Triage is a method to prioritize patients:

- **Red Tag**: Life-threatening neuro symptoms (unconscious, no response, major head injury)
- **Yellow Tag**: Serious but stable symptoms (confused speech, minor seizures, vomiting)
- **Green Tag**: Walking wounded
- **Black Tag**: Deceased or unsurvivable injuries

First Aid Priorities

- **Do not move** victims unless safe.
- Focus first on those with:
    - Unconsciousness
    - Seizures
    - Severe bleeding from the head
    - Difficulty breathing
- Assign bystanders to:

    - Apply pressure to bleeding
    - Support neck and head
    - Comfort conscious patients

Disaster Readiness Kits Should Include

- Stretcher/sheets
- Torch
- Cold packs
- CPR mask
- Rope, blankets
- Symptom cards for stroke/seizure
- Basic medication (as per trained personnel)

Chapter 18

Role of Telemedicine in Neurological Emergencies

The New Era of Virtual Neurology

With technology advancing, **telemedicine** has become a valuable tool to manage emergencies when doctors are not physically available.

Benefits in Neurological First Aid

- **Remote guidance** from neurologists to paramedics or laypersons.
- **Video assessment** of stroke signs.
- **Decision support** for seizure or fainting cases.
- Faster **referral and transport decisions.**

Tele-Neuro Tools

- **Mobile apps** with stroke/epilepsy management checklists.
- **Wearable alert systems** for seizure-prone individuals.
- **Smart watches** with fall detection and pulse tracking.
- Community centers with **telehealth kiosks.**

Limitations

- Requires stable internet connectivity.
- Cannot replace physical first aid—only supports it.

Chapter 19

Preventing Neurological Emergencies - Public Health and Education

Why Prevention is the Best First Aid

Most neurological emergencies are **either preventable** or **can be caught early** with awareness and routine care.

Stroke Prevention

- **Control blood pressure**, diabetes, and cholesterol.
- Avoid smoking, excess alcohol, and junk food.
- **Daily physical activity and regular health checkups.**

Injury Prevention

- **Wear helmets** while riding two-wheelers.
- **Use seatbelts** in cars.
- **Childproof homes** to prevent falls.
- Install **anti-slip mats** in bathrooms for elderly.
- Train in **safe lifting and handling** to avoid spinal injuries.

Seizure Management Awareness

- Know **first aid steps.**
- Keep schools and public places **seizure-ready** with staff training.
- Carry **ID cards or medical bracelets** for seizure-prone individuals.

Public Awareness Campaigns

- Organize "**Brain Health Days**" in schools, colleges, workplaces.
- Display **stroke and seizure posters** in clinics, bus stands, railway stations.
- Use **local language videos** and **radio shows** for wider reach.

Key Takeaways from Part IV

Situation	Recommended Action
Rural Area	Use improvised tools, stabilize, transport cautiously
Mass Casualty	Use triage, prioritize breathing + consciousness
Telemedicine	Use video calls and apps for remote guidance
Prevention	Promote helmet use, BP control, elder safety
Public Education	Posters, sessions, kits, health camps

Appendix A

Neurological Emergency First Aid Checklist

	Step
1	Ensure the scene is safe for both rescuer and patient
2	Check responsiveness: Tap and shout
3	Call for emergency medical services (EMS)
4	Check for breathing and pulse
5	Place patient in recovery position if unconscious but breathing
6	Use FAST assessment for stroke
7	Time the duration of seizures
8	Avoid giving anything by mouth
9	Support head and neck if spinal injury is suspected
10	Record signs, symptoms, and time of onset

Appendix B

Sample Neurological Symptoms Diary Sheet

Use this to track symptoms during or after an episode.

Time	Event	Symptoms Observed	Actions Taken	Response
2:05 pm	Fall	Unconscio us for 1 min	Recovery position, called EMS	Regained consciousne ss
3:30 pm	Seizur e	Shaking, frothing, 3 min	Protected head, turned sideways	Drowsy afterward

Appendix C
Emergency Contact Template

Post this sheet in a visible location:

- **Name of Patient:**
- **Date of Birth:**
- **Known Conditions:** (e.g., epilepsy, high BP)
- **Medications:**
- **Blood Group:**
- **Primary Contact Name:**
- **Phone:**
- **Secondary Contact Name:**
- **Doctor's Name:**
- **Nearest Hospital:**

Appendix D
FAST Assessment Form

Use when stroke is suspected.

Test	What to Do	Observation	Normal/ Abnormal
Face	Ask the person to smile	Left side droops	Abnormal
Arms	Ask to raise both arms	Right arm drifts	Abnormal
Speech	Ask to repeat a sentence	Slurred	Abnormal
Time	Note time symptoms started	4:45 pm	—

Appendix E
CPR and BLS Flowcharts

For Adults

1. **Unresponsive** → Check for breathing/pulse
2. **No breathing/pulse** → Call EMS → Start **30 compressions + 2 breaths**
3. **Use AED** as soon as available
4. Continue until help arrives or signs of life return

For Children

1. Start with **5 initial breaths**, then **30:2 compressions : breaths**
2. Continue for 1 minute before calling EMS if alone

Appendix F
Pupil Check Reference Chart

Condition	Pupil Reaction	Possible Indication
Normal	Equal and reactive	Healthy brain activity
Unequal pupils	One dilated, one normal	Possible brain injury
Fixed & dilated	No reaction to light	Severe brain damage or death
Sluggish response	Slow constriction	Pressure/injury in brain

Appendix G

Neurological Emergency Kit Essentials

Item	Purpose
Gloves, masks	Infection control
CPR mask	Rescue breathing
Cold packs	Migraine, fever
Flashlight	Pupil check
Emergency ID card	Medical details
Clean towel	Head support, bleeding
Timer/watch	Seizure duration
Basic medications (as prescribed)	Symptom management

Glossary of Key Terms

- **Aphasia**: Inability to speak or understand language
- **Ataxia**: Loss of coordination or balance
- **Hemiplegia**: Paralysis of one side of the body
- **Postictal state**: Recovery phase after a seizure
- **Ischemia**: Lack of blood flow
- **Glasgow Coma Scale (GCS)**: A scoring system to assess consciousness
- **Cerebellum**: Brain region for balance and coordination
- **Seizure aura**: A sensory warning sign before a seizure begins

References and Further Reading

- World Health Organization. **Neurological Disorders: Public Health Challenges**
- American Stroke Association. **FAST Stroke Recognition Tool**
- International League Against Epilepsy (ILAE) Guidelines
- National Institute of Neurological Disorders and Stroke (NINDS)
- Advanced First Aid Manuals (Red Cross, St. John Ambulance)

Summary of Appendices

Practical Tools for Real-Life Use

Tool	Use
First Aid Checklist	Quick steps for emergencies
Symptom Diary	Helps in hospital communication
Contact Card	Ensures immediate access to vital info
FAST Form	Stroke recognition and documentation
Flowcharts	Visual guides for CPR/BLS
Pupil Chart	Assess neurological damage
Emergency Kit List	Prepare and personalize kits

List of Published Books

1. Gupta K and Jain M. Vridhopayogi Vyanjan: Vridhjano ke liye Upcharatmak Pak Vidhiyan. Abhinav Prakashan. Ajmer. 2016. ISBN: 978-938418946-4

2. Gupta K. Community Science and Sustainable Community Development. Lambart Academic Publication. Germany 2021. ISBN: 978-620419757-9

3. Gupta K. 75 years of Indian Independence: Food and Nutritional Achievements, Opportunities and Challenges (Volume 1). Notion Press. Chennai. 2022. ISBN: 979-888883053-6

4. Gupta K. 75 years of Indian Independence: Food and Nutritional Achievements, Opportunities and Challenges (Volume 2). Notion Press. Chennai. 2022. ISBN: 979-888883757-3

5. Gupta K. 75 years of Indian Independence: Food and Nutritional Achievements, Opportunities and Challenges (Volume 3). Notion Press. Chennai. 2022. ISBN: 979-888909005-2

6. Gupta K. Aazadi ka Amrit Mahotsav: Community Science Achievements, Opportunities and Challenges. BlueRose One Publishers. India. 2023. ISBN: 978-935704938-2

7. Gupta K. Nutrition Education: An Important Pillar of Health. Notion Press. Chennai. 2023. ISBN: 979-888959915-9

8. Gupta K, Bhushan V, Pandey A. Issues with Girls. Notion Press. Chennai. 2023. ISBN: 979-889026221-9

9. Gupta K, Tripathi KM, Meena N, Sukhwal I, Soni V. Recent Trends in Community Science. BlueRose One Publishers. India. 2023. ISBN: 978-935819026-7

10. Gupta K, Katiyar P, Meena S, Tripathi KM,. Millets: The Miracle of Nature. Notion Press. Chennai. 2023. ISBN: 979-889066606-2

11. Gupta K, Cherian B, Ramalakshmi, Harjai K. Health and Wellness (A basic guide to obtain good health). Notion Press. Chennai. 2023. ISBN: 979-889067222-3

12. Gupta K, Gaur V, Kumari R, Mishra S, Arya L, Mukharjee G. Health for All. Notion Press. Chennai. 2023. ISBN: 979-889133024-5

13. Gupta K, Swamy D, Jain S, Sangeeta, Rochani C, Verma R. Current Advances in Community Science. Notion Press. Chennai. 2023. ISBN: 979-889186087-2

14. Gupta K, Katiyar P, Verma P, Pawar RV, Sangeeta. Food Safety & Security- A Basic Guide. Notion Press. Chennai. 2023. ISBN: 979-889233007-7

15. Gupta K, Venkatappa KG, Devi KV, Sangeeta, Pal P. Brain: Associations, Wellness & Treatment. Notion Press. Chennai. 2024. ISBN: 979-889233671-0

16. Gupta K, Mukharjee G, Esaivani KB, Sangeeta, Anuradha K, Jethwani P. Handbook on Inflammatory Bowel Disease (Volume 1). Hemakshee Publication. Sikar. 2024. ISBN: 978-81-969920-0-2

17. Gupta K, Annapurna A, Verma P, Pal P, Supriya. Nurturing Bonds: A Holistic Guide to Breastfeeding Bliss. Hemakshee Publication. Sikar. 2024. ISBN: 978-81-969920-3-3.

18. Gupta K, Das B, Deep EMS, Supriya, Singh S, Singhal AK. Handbook on Inflammatory Bowel Disease (Volume 2). Hemakshee Publication. Sikar. 2024. ISBN: 978-81-969920-1-9

19. Gupta K, Supriya, Annapurna A, Sangeeta, Marwaha P. Nourishing Bonds: A Comprehensive Guide to Weaning. Hemakshee Publication. Sikar. 2024. ISBN: 978-81-971773-3-0.

20. Gupta K, Bajpai A, Verma P, Pal P, Singh T, Singh J. Skill Inculcation and Sustainable Community Development. Hemakshee Publication. Sikar. 2024. ISBN: 978-81-971773-7-8.

21. Gupta K, Tiwari T, Singh K,, Venkatappa KG, Chaturvedi B, Sangeeta. Empowering Future-

Skill Inculcation and Sustainable Communities. Hemakshee Publication. Sikar. 2024. ISBN: 978-81-971773-4-7.

22. Gupta K, Gunjan G, Vernekar GK, Mukharjee G, Sangeeta, Babu VS. Handbook on Inflammatory Bowel Disease (Volume 3). Hemakshee Publication. Sikar. 2024. ISBN: 978-81-978907-0-3

23. Gupta K. Golden Guidelines for Optimizing Elderly Nutrition. Hemakshee Publication. Sikar. 2024. ISBN: 978-81-976151-3-9

24. Gupta K, Supriya, Srivastava S, Saraswat M, Srivastava D, Sangeeta. Harmony in Diversity-Integrating Food, Textiles and Human Development in Communities. Hemakshee Publication. Sikar. 2024. ISBN: 978-81-978907-2-7.

25. Gupta K, Mukherjee G, Deep EMS, Sangeeta, Kondle VK. Soulful Serenity: Yoga and Meditation for Blissful Life. Hemakshee Publication. Sikar. 2024. ISBN: 978-93-48873-86-6.

26. Gupta K, Tiwari N, Aherkar J, Venkatappa KG, Sharma P, Ganguly B. Holistic Horizon: Integrating Knowledge for Sustainable Communities Hemakshee Publication. Sikar. 2024. ISBN: 978-81-978907-4-1.

27. Gupta K, Vernekar GK, Padma L, Verma P, Mishra S, Tiwari N. Celiac Disease- From Pathophysiology to Patient Care (Volume 1). Hemakshee Publication. Sikar. 2025. ISBN: 978-93-48873-99-6

28. Gupta K, Avhad SS, Kondle VK, Vernekar GK, Kumar S, Sangeeta. Celiac Disease- From Pathophysiology to Patient Care (Volume 2). Hemakshee Publication. Sikar. 2025. ISBN: 978-93-48873-79-8

29. Gupta K, Agrawal D, Gupta S, Gupta S. From Debt to Wealth: Your Journey to Financial Freedom in India. Hemakshee Publication. Sikar. 2025. ISBN: 978-93-48873-74-3

30. Gupta K, Jain T, Mahajan S, Yadav AR, Babu VS, Vernekar, GK. Celiac Disease- Insights and Innovations (Volume 1). Hemakshee Publication. Sikar. 2025. ISBN: 978-93-48873-94-1

31. Gupta K, Supriya, Vernekar, GK, Jha A, Anuradha K. Celiac Disease- Insights and Innovations (Volume 2). Hemakshee Publication. Sikar. 2025. ISBN: 978-93-48873-45-3

Note: These books are available on publisher's website, Amazon and FlipKart

www.ingramcontent.com/pod-product-compliance
Ingram Content Group UK Ltd.
Pitfield, Milton Keynes, MK11 3LW, UK
UKHW021341190726
13845UKWH00027B/671